SUGAR FREE RECIPES

Speedy and Easy 30 MINUTE Sugar Free Recipes for Breakfast, Lunch, Dinner, and Dessert

Gina Crawford

Evita Publishing, PO Box 306, Station A, Vancouver Island, BC V9W 5B1 Canada

Table of Contents

Introduction

Sugar is such a common ingredient in our food today that it's often hard to find anything that doesn't contain sugar. Many recipes include sugar in one form or another even if the recipe appears perfectly pure and healthy.

When I got determined to turn my health around, it became very important for me to live a sugar free life. I started by taking sugar out of my existing recipes, but that made the food taste bland and boring. Not a welcome change for the sugar monster inside of me.

The more I tried to stick with bland, boring, unsweetened eating, the more my sugar monster grew. Eventually, my gnawing desire for sugar led to an inevitable, out of control late night sugar binge that left me feeling guilty for weeks afterward.

In a desperate attempt to kick sugar out of my life for good, I decided to explore the world of sugar free recipes. I was SO glad that I did! They made a world of difference!

I absolutely fell in love with the fact that I could eat sugar free without sacrificing taste!

In this book, I will share my favorite sugar free breakfast, lunch, dinner, and dessert recipes with you. I've provided a wide variety of recipes that will allow you to eat sugar free for quite a while.

Sugar can be as addictive as a drug, so the fact that you are taking the steps necessary to rid yourself of sugar is commendable.

I hope you enjoy the recipes!

Chapter 1

BREAKFAST

When diet is wrong, medicine is of no use.
When diet is correct, medicine is of no need.
– Ayurvedic Proverb

Eggs Nested in Shiitake Mushrooms and Sautéed Chard

Shiitake mushrooms have been a symbol of longevity in Asia for years because of their amazing health-promoting properties. In fact, the Chinese have used Shiitake's medicinally for more than 6000 years. Shiitake's are an excellent source of iron and copper, they support the immune and cardiovascular system, and they have a natural ability to ward off inflammation.

Chard contains 13 different antioxidants and is a great source of fiber and protein. It also contains a phytonutrient called betalains which has an anti-inflammatory and detoxifying effect on the body.

Ingredients

Extra virgin olive oil.....2 tablespoons

Yellow onion..... ½ cup chopped

Fresh chard.....½ pound sliced (separate the chard ribs from the leaves)

Shiitake mushrooms.....3 large, sliced into 1/4-inch slices

Eggs.....2 medium or large

Salt.....to taste

Black pepper.....to taste

Directions

Add olive oil to a medium saucepan and heat.

Add the onions, chard ribs, and mushrooms. Sauté on medium heat for five minutes or until the onions turn opaque.

Add the chard leaves to the saucepan. Toss with tongs or use a spatula to ensure all the ingredients are mixed together well. When thoroughly mixed, spread over the bottom of the pan evenly.

Add one or two eggs to the center of the pan. This creates the nest. Reduce heat to medium low and cook the eggs for 3-4 minutes. Remove from heat when the eggs have cooked through. Transfer to a serving plate. Serve.

Sugar Free Cheesy Egg Muffins

Half-and half is a good source of vitamin A. Vitamin A supports the immune system and vision. When we obtain vitamin A from animal sources we are obtaining the retinoid form of vitamin A. The retinoid form is important for pregnancy, childbirth, infancy, and child growth. For adults, it is important for night vision, red blood cell production, heart health, and resistance to infectious diseases.

Ingredients

Half and half.....8 fluid ounces

Eggs.....12 large

Mozzarella cheese.....¾ cup, shredded

Parmesan cheese.....½ cup, shredded

Green onion.....¾ cup, finely chopped

Black pepper.....to taste

Salt.....to taste

Directions

Preheat oven to 400 °F (200 °C).

Combine all the ingredients in a medium bowl.

In a muffin pan, add muffin paper cups and spoon the mixture into the cups. Stir periodically since the ingredients will separate.

Cook until golden brown, about 20 minutes.

Creamy Stuffed Eggs with Avocado

Avocados have numerous health benefits. They support heart and eye health, lower cholesterol levels, control blood pressure, reduce the risk of stroke, protect against cancer, fight free radicals, reduce the risk of inflammatory and degenerative disorders etc.

Eggs are also full of an array of nutrients. They contain numerous vitamins including potassium, vitamin A, and many B vitamins, and they are a beneficial source of protein and healthy fat.

Ingredients

Eggs.....6 large, hard-boiled

White vinegar.....2 teaspoons

Avocado.....¼ cup puréed

Dash of salt and black pepper

Dash of nutmeg (optional)

Directions

Peel the shell off the hard-boiled eggs and rinse.

Cut the eggs in half lengthwise.

Remove the egg yolks and place them in a small bowl.

On a platter, place the egg whites in a circle and set to the side.

Add vinegar, puréed avocado, salt, and black pepper to the egg yolks.

Using a fork, mix all the ingredients together until the egg yolks are smooth and forming a creamy texture.

Spoon the creamy mixture into each of the egg whites and place on a serving platter.

Sprinkle the eggs with nutmeg and serve immediately, or wrap them with plastic and refrigerate for later.

Rise and Shine Morning Meatballs

Using fat-free cheddar cheese and lean pork sausage in this recipe will help to reduce the fat content, and make this low carbohydrate meaty dish a real winner!

Makes 50 to 60 meatballs

Ingredients

Fat-free cheddar cheese..... ½ pound, shredded

Eggs.....3 large

Lean pork sausage.....32 ounces

Yellow onion.....2 tablespoons, minced

Lean ground beef.....1 pound

Black pepper.....to taste

Directions

Preheat the oven to 350 °F (175 °C).

Stir all the ingredients together in a medium bowl. Add pepper to taste.

Mix thoroughly and form into 1 ½ inch balls.

Place the meatballs on a baking sheet that has rims so that the drippings remain in the pan.

Bake 18-20 minutes. Serve.

Tip: If you are interested in making an extra batch of breakfast meatballs for later, the meatballs freeze well, so feel free to freeze as many as you like!

Banana Cinnamon Pancakes

Potassium is a mineral that acts as an electrolyte. Common electrolytes are sodium, potassium, bicarbonate, and chloride. We need the right balance of potassium and sodium to stay active and feel energized. Bananas are a great source of potassium. Potassium is also required for keeping the heart, muscle tissue, brain, kidneys, and other vital organ systems in good shape.

Ingredients

Banana.....1 medium or large

Egg.....1 medium or large

Sea salt.....1 teaspoon

Cinnamon.....1 teaspoon

Whole wheat flour.....½ teaspoon

Extra virgin olive oil.....2 tablespoons

Fresh raspberries, blackberries, strawberries

Pure maple syrup

Directions

In a small bowl, mash the banana with a fork.

Add egg, cinnamon, wheat flour, and salt to the bowl.

Mix the ingredients together to form pancake batter.

Preheat the extra virgin olive oil in a skillet over low to medium heat.

Scoop the batter onto the pan using a large spoon or a measuring cup.

Watch for bubbles to form from the center of the pancake.

When the edges have formed a crispy ring, flip the pancake over and cook until nicely brown.

Remove from skillet and plate.

Top with fresh raspberries, blackberries, or strawberries and pure maple syrup.

Raspberry Oatmeal Swirl

Steel cut oats are the least processed type of oat cereal. They are whole grain groats (inner portion of the oat kernel) that have been chopped into sesame seed sized chunks.

Raspberries are power-packed with antioxidants, phytonutrients, vitamins, fiber, iron, magnesium, potassium, zinc, etc. They prevent damage to DNA cells from free radicals and improve vision, immunity, increase blood formation, and promote weight loss.

Ingredients

Steel cut oats.....1 cup

Water.....3 cups

Salt.....pinch

Sugar free raspberry preserves.....2 tablespoons

Sugar free whipped topping.....2 tablespoons

Directions

Pour the water into a pot and bring to a boil. Stir in the salt and oats.

Bring the water back up to a boil then reduce to medium-low heat.

Simmer the oats with the lid ajar stirring frequently for 25 minutes.

When oats are ready, place them in a bowl. Add sugar free raspberry preserves and sugar free whipped topping. Serve warm.

Sweet Treat Breakfast Omelet

Coconut is referred to as a miracle fruit and "superfood" due to its health benefits and healing properties. One of the reasons it is so amazing is because it contains a unique combination of fatty acids that have a profound effect on our health.

Vanilla extract is made from vanilla beans that are pods, or fruits, grown on tropical climbing orchids. Vanilla has long been used for its medicinal properties by Mayan and Aztec civilizations because it contains anti-inflammatory and anti-carcinogenic properties that act as cancer cell inhibitors.

Ingredients

Eggs.....2 whole eggs, beaten

Vanilla extract.....1 teaspoon

Coconut oil.....1 tablespoon

Directions

In a small bowl, add the eggs and vanilla. Beat with a fork until well mixed.

Heat the coconut oil in a small skillet over medium heat. Add the egg mixture to the pan. Tilt the pan until the egg covers the bottom of the skillet evenly.

Cook the eggs until firmly set with no visible liquid remaining. Fold the eggs over. Plate and serve warm.

8 things to serve with your sweet treat breakfast omelet (all optional):

1 - Toasted almonds, lemon curd, and honey

2 - Nut butters such as almond and macadamia

3 - Fresh fruit such as banana, apple, and strawberries

4 - Lemon curd as a filling

5 - A dollop of yogurt or sour cream

6 - A dollop of whipped coconut cream

7 - Sprinkle of cinnamon

8 - Chopped pecans

Nutty Pumpkin Porridge

Pepitas is the Spanish culinary word for shelled pumpkin seeds. Pumpkin seeds are packed with manganese, phosphorus, copper, magnesium, zinc, protein, and iron. In fact, one quarter cup of pumpkin seeds provides almost half the daily recommended amount of magnesium. Pumpkin seeds also contain antioxidants that search out and destroy free radicals. The antioxidants are contained in the seed as well as the shell. Pumpkin seeds have long been associated with men's health due to their high zinc content which supports prostrate health.

Ingredients

Shredded unsweetened coconut.....¼ cup

Raw walnuts.....¼ cup

Sliced almonds.....¼ cup

Raw shelled pumpkin seeds.....2 tablespoons

Flaxseed meal.....1 tablespoon

Hot water.....½ cup

Honey.....½ tablespoon, or to taste (optional)

Directions

In a food processor, add coconut, walnuts, almonds, pumpkin seeds, and flaxseed meal. Mix until finely ground.

Boil water in a medium saucepan.

In a microwave-safe bowl, add the boiling water and honey. Stir.

Add the ground nut mix to the water and honey mixture. Stir until mixed.

Place the microwave-safe bowl into the microwave and cook for 30 seconds.

Stir again and serve immediately.

To cook on stovetop:

Heat over medium-low heat for 4-5 minutes.

Stir during cooking time and serve warm.

Easy Sugar Free Granola

This is a nice, easy recipe for sugar free granola. The rolled oats are the main ingredient for this recipe. All the other ingredients in the recipe depend on your taste preference. The rolled oats high fiber content helps to remove cholesterol from the digestive system that could potentially end up in your blood stream.

Ingredients

Chopped dates.....1 cup

Water.....1 cup

Roller oats.....8 cups

Chopped walnuts.....½ cup

Raisins.....1 cup

Wheat germ.....1 cup

Sunflower seeds.....½ cup

Slivered almonds.....½ cup

Shredded unsweetened coconut.....2 cups

Vegetable oil.....¼ cup

Frozen apple juice..... ¼ cup thawed

Directions

Preheat oven to 350 °F (175 °C).

In a small saucepan, on medium heat, add the water and dates.

Cook until the water and dates form a thick mixture or paste like substance. Remove from heat. Set aside.

In a large bowl, add rolled oats, walnuts, wheat germ, raisins, sunflower seeds, almonds, and coconut. Take this mixture and spread a thin layer over a baking sheet. You may need to repeat this step in batches if your baking sheet is small.

Bake for 7 minutes then remove from oven. Transfer to the bowl of date paste then add the apple concentrate and oil to the bowl. Mix ingredients together and return to the baking sheet. Bake an additional 7-10 minutes. Stir occasionally until lightly brown.

Granola will become crisper as it cools. Store in an airtight container.

Breakfast Salmon and Fennel Salad

Recent studies suggest that the protein and amino acid content in salmon called bioactive peptides may provide more nutrients for joint cartilage, insulin effectiveness, and digestive tract inflammation than once suspected.

Fennel has many health benefits including relief from anemia, indigestion, and respiratory disorders.

Ingredients

Pink salmon.....2 tins, 213 grams each

Fennel.....finely sliced (all parts of the fennel are edible so it is only a matter of preference here)

Spring onions.....2 stalks, finely sliced

Broccoli florets.....3 heads, sliced

Brown rice.....½ cup

Parsley.....fresh (to taste)

Water.....1 cup

Fresh lime juice & cracked black pepper to taste (optional)

Directions

In a steamer, add the water and then the broccoli florets. Bring the water to a boil and steam the broccoli until cooked. About 7 minutes. Remove from heat. Rinse in cold water then set aside.

In a medium bowl, add the pink salmon, fennel, spring onions, and broccoli.

In a medium saucepan, add one part brown rice to two parts water. You do not need too much rice added as this is only providing texture to the dish. One cup of water to 1/2 cup of rice is more than enough for both cans of salmon.

Mix all the ingredients together. Add lime and black pepper to taste.

Serve chilled.

Broccoli Zucchini Egg Bake

Broccoli is a cruciferous vegetable that should be eaten several times a week. Its many health benefits include kidney, immune system, and heart health as well as the prevention of arthritis and cancer. Broccoli also contains Vitamin K which supports bone health and prevents blood from clotting and Vitamin C which helps fight against free radicals.

Makes 6 servings

Ingredients

Eggs.....8 medium

White onion.....½ large, diced

Zucchini.....2 medium, diced

Broccoli.....1 medium head, chopped

Salt.....1 teaspoon

Black pepper.....½ teaspoon

Fresh parsley.....1 tablespoon, chopped

Directions

Preheat the oven to 350 °F (175 °C).

On a cutting board, prepare the zucchini and broccoli

In a small bowl, add the eggs, salt and pepper then whisk together.

Add the zucchini and broccoli to the bowl of eggs.

Stir to coat the vegetables with the egg mixture.

Coat a ramekin or a single serving baking dish with coconut oil non-stick spray and pour the mixture into the baking dish.

Bake the prepared dish for 25 minutes or until the eggs are set.

Remove the dish from the oven and let it rest for 5 minutes before topping with chopped parsley. Serve warm.

Yum!

Bacon Wrapped Omelet Mini's

These tasty little omelet bites are packed with protein and flavor. Chicken is rich in a mineral called selenium that helps prevent arthritis. Chicken is also a great stress reliever because it contains vitamin B5 or pantothenic acid which has a calming effect on the nerves. It is also a great source of lean protein that contains little fat.

Ingredients

Chicken.....2 cups, diced and cooked

Bacon.....12 thin slices

Eggs.....4 large

Egg whites.....12 large

Spinach.....2 cups, chopped

Green pepper.....½ medium, chopped

Red pepper.....½ medium, chopped

Non-stick cooking spray

Directions

Preheat the oven to 350°F (175 °C).

Cook the bacon in a pan over medium high heat until it is cooked through. Make sure it doesn't get crispy, about 5 minutes.

Spray a muffin tin with non-stick cooking spray then wrap one piece of bacon around the outer edges of each tin.

In a medium sized bowl, scramble the four large eggs with the twelve egg whites. Add the red and green peppers, diced chicken, and spinach. Season with salt and pepper.

Combine the mixture and pour it into each muffin tin lined with bacon. Use a spoon or ladle to transfer the mixture.

Bake until the eggs are fluffy and slightly browned on top, about 25 minutes.

Tip: You can top this dish with avocado or change things up by adding different ingredients like mushrooms, onions, or sausage.

Sugar Free Chicken and Bacon Breakfast Burrito

This breakfast burrito is jam-packed with protein and antioxidants. It's also dairy-free, grain-free, soy-free, nut-free, gluten-free, and of course, sugar-free! It will give you a blast of energy to start your day!

Ingredients

Sliced ham.....1-2 slices (select a ham that is big enough to fold and has a medium thickness)

Eggs.....2 (you can use egg whites only if you like)

Spinach..... ¼ cup, chopped

Black olives..... ¼ cup, sliced

Red bell pepper..... ¼ finely chopped

Tomato..... ¼ cup, chopped

Extra virgin olive oil.....2 tablespoons

Salsa

Guacamole

Cilantro.....chopped, to taste

Directions

Heat the oil in a skillet over medium high heat.

Add all the vegetables and sauté them.

Whisk the eggs in a small bowl and add them to the pan

Scramble and mix until thoroughly cooked.

Remove the egg/vegetable mixture. Take a slice of ham and place some of the egg mixture on it. Chop the cilantro and sprinkle some of it on top of the egg mixture. Roll the ham slice around the cilantro egg mixture and place it on the skillet to grill until the ham is slightly brown on each side.

Serve with salsa and guacamole.

Guilt-Free Eggs Benedict

Tomatoes are primarily known for their impressive antioxidant content, including their rich concentration of lycopene. Lycopene is a more effective antioxidant than other carotenoids such as beta-carotene. Its powerful antioxidant actions help to maintain strong cell membranes that protect cells. Strong, healthy cell membranes play a vital role in the prevention of many diseases.

Ingredients

Tomato.....2 cut into thick slices (half inch thick)

Avocado.....½ peeled and pitted (cut the avocado into 3 sections)

Eggs.....2 large

Salt.....1 teaspoon

White vinegar.....2 teaspoons

Hollandaise sauce:

Egg yolks.....2

1 % Greek yogurt.....½ cup, plain

Lemon juice.....½ tablespoon

Butter.....1 tablespoon, melted

Sea salt.....½-1 teaspoon

Directions

In a small saucepan, bring 1 to 2 inches of water to a boil then lower the heat to a low simmer. Add salt and vinegar.

Crack one egg into a small cup. Using a wooden spoon, stir the water to create a whirlpool effect. Drop the egg into the center of the water whirlpool.

Cook for 3 minutes and remove the egg with a slotted spoon when the egg whites have set. Transfer to a side dish, keep warm, and repeat with the second egg. Remove the second egg and place on the side dish.

Hollandaise sauce directions:

Using the same saucepan (with the water still at a low simmer), place a stainless steel bowl larger than the sauce pan on the rim of the pan but not touching the boiling water.

Whisk yolks in the bowl until the mixture looks about double in volume. Drizzle in the butter and continue to whisk until combined.

Stir in the yogurt and lemon juice and heat through. Add salt to taste.

Top with freshly ground pepper and hot sauce if desired.

Plating:

Place 1 slice of tomato on a plate.

Lay the three avocado slices on top of the tomato.

Place one egg on top of the avocado slices.

Top with hollandaise sauce.

Enjoy!

Chapter 2

LUNCH

Healthy eating is a way of life, so it's important to establish routines that are simple, realistic, and ultimately livable.

– Arthur Agatston

Dijon Broccoli Chicken

Dijon mustard uses a brown mustard seed called brassica juncea. There are over 40 types of mustard plants. Mustard plants are in the same family as cruciferous vegetables like broccoli, Brussels sprouts, and cabbage. Three of the 40 mustard plants are where we get our mustard seeds for the production of mustard.

There is the black mustard seed, which is most pungent and the white mustard seed. The white mustard seed is actually yellow in color but lighter than the brown mustard seed used in Dijon mustards. Mustards are full of selenium, omega-3 fats, manganese, phosphorus, magnesium, copper, and vitamin B1.

Ingredients

Chicken breast.....1 pound, sliced into thin strips

Extra virgin olive oil.....1 ½ tablespoons

Chicken broth.....½ cup

Soy sauce.....2 tablespoons

Broccoli florets.....4 cups

Dijon mustard.....6 teaspoons

Garlic clove.....1 minced

Directions

Combine the chicken broth and soy sauce in a small bowl. Stir so that the chicken is nicely covered in the soy sauce. Set aside.

Heat the olive oil in a large skillet on medium heat. Add the garlic and broccoli. Cook the broccoli until it is crisp on the outside yet tender on the inside. Remove the broccoli from the skillet and cover.

Add the chicken (only) to the skillet and cook until it is crispy and cooked through. Reserve the sauce.

Add the sauce (chicken broth and soy sauce mixture) to the chicken.

Bring to a boil then reduce the heat to medium low.

Add the mustard and stir well to mix.

Return the broccoli to the skillet and stir to mix. Cook until heated through. Serve warm.

Mint Chicken Burgers

Mint chicken burgers are great hot or cold. Make them warm one night and serve them up cold for lunch the next day. Eating a variety of spices and herbs are a necessary part of any diet. This recipe's got you covered and provides a nice tasty blend of each.

Serves 4

Ingredients

Ground chicken.....500 grams

Coriander.....½ cup, finely chopped

Mint.....½ cup, finely chopped

Ground cumin.....1 teaspoon

Sweet paprika.....1 teaspoon

Red chili.....1 finely diced

Garlic clove.....1 minced

Gluten-free breadcrumbs.....2 tablespoons

Egg.....1 (to bind)

Sea salt.....to taste

Ground black pepper.....to taste

Coconut oil.....1 tablespoon

Whole grain burger buns.....4

Directions

In a large bowl, add the chicken, coriander, mint, cumin, paprika, red chili, garlic, and breadcrumbs. Stir well mixing the ingredients together. Add an egg and mix well.

Form four chicken patties and place in the refrigerator for 20 minutes to chill and firm.

In a large frying pan, add a tablespoon of coconut oil over medium heat.

Fry the burgers for 4-5 minutes on each side.

Chicken burgers should cook all the way through with a golden brown crispy texture on each side.

Serve with your favorite toppings on a whole grain burger bun.

Low-Carb Turkey and Egg Lettuce Wraps

While this recipe is certainly versatile, using romaine lettuce will give you an added nutritional boost when it comes to a lettuce wrap. Two cups of romaine lettuce will give you 107 percent of your daily vitamin K allowance, 45.5 percent of your vitamin A allowance, and 31.9 percent folate. These wraps are also an excellent, low-carb snack.

Ingredients

Romaine lettuce.....8 medium lettuce leaves

Nitrate-free deli-style turkey.....8 slices

Eggs.....8 large, boiled

Directions

In a medium pot, add all eight eggs and cover with water.

Turn the heat to high and boil the eggs for 10 minutes.

Remove pot from heat and run cold water over the hard-boiled eggs.

Peel the eggs.

Take the eight lettuce leaves and wash them under cold running water

Place a lettuce leaf on a serving plate and add a slice of deli style turkey on top of it. Cut a hard-boiled egg into slices and place the slices on top of the turkey.

Roll the lettuce leaf with the turkey and egg to form a wrap. Serve.

Broccoli Rabe Pesto with Fresh Basil

Broccoli Rabe is not broccoli rather it is more like a mustard green, or turnip green. It is commonly referred to as Rabe pronounced Rob. Rabe is a great source of calcium, vitamin K, folate, and antioxidants.

Ingredients

Parmesan cheese......6 tablespoons, shredded

Fresh basil....20 leaves

Extra virgin olive oil......1/3 cup

Lemon.....1 juiced

Broccoli rabe.....8 ounces

Garlic.....3 teaspoons

Slivered almonds.....¼ cup

Directions

Fill a medium saucepan half full of water. Bring water to a boil and add the broccoli rabe. Boil for 3 minutes.

While the broccoli rabe is boiling, prepare a medium bowl of ice water.

When the rabe has boiled the full 3 minutes, remove it from the heat and strain. Transfer the rabe from the strainer straight to the bowl of ice water to stop the cooking process.

Next, transfer the rabe to the food processor. Add the garlic, parmesan cheese, basil, lemon, and almonds. Pulse the processor several times, then drizzle the olive oil in and scrape the sides. Pulse a few more times then season with salt and pepper.

The mixture is great as a spread for Melba toast, toasted pita chips, or mixed in hot pasta.

Mango Salsa

Cilantro is a powerful, natural cleansing herb. It is effective for toxic metal cleansing because the chemical compounds in cilantro bind with toxic metals and separate them from the tissue.

Mangos are a great source of omega-3 and omega-6. The mango also provides carotenoids, polyphenols, phytochemicals, and antioxidants.

Ingredients

Roma tomatoes.....2 cups, diced

Mango.....1 ½ cups, diced

Onion.....½ cup, diced

Cilantro..... ½ cup, chopped

Fresh lime juice.....2 tablespoons

Cider vinegar.....1 tablespoon

Salt..... ½ teaspoon

Black pepper.....½ teaspoon

Garlic.....2 cloves, minced

Stevia.....2-3 drops to taste

Directions

In a large bowl, add the roma tomatoes, mangos, onions, and cilantro. Mix together with a large spoon or spatula.

In a small bowl, add the stevia, lime juice, cider vinegar, salt, pepper, and minced garlic cloves. Whisk the ingredients together then drizzle it over the tomato and mango mixture.

Serve immediately or wrap with plastic and refrigerate to chill and serve later.

Southwest Salsa

Did you know that corn stabilizes the macronutrients in our digestive system, which helps to prevent our digestive track from digesting too rapidly or even too slowly? This process also prevents blood sugar from spiking or dropping by leveling the digestive process with sufficient levels of fiber and protein.

Ingredients

Yellow corn.....1-15 ounce can, drained

White corn.....1-15 ounce can, drained

Black beans.....2-15 ounce cans, drained and rinsed

Italian style diced tomatoes.....1-14.5 ounce can, drained

Cilantro.....1 bunch, finely chopped

Green onions.....5 stalks

Red onion.....1 small, finely chopped

Red bell pepper.....1 seeded and chopped

Garlic.....1 tablespoon, minced

Lime juice.....¼ cup

Avocado.....1 peeled, pitted, and diced

Extra virgin olive oil.....2 tablespoons

Directions

In a large bowl, add the yellow corn, white corn, black beans, tomatoes, cilantro, green onions, red onions, bell pepper, and garlic.

Stir the mixture gently while slowly adding the lime juice.

Dice half the avocado and stir it into the mixture. Next, cut the other half of the avocado into slices and decorate the top of the mixture with it.

Drizzle the olive oil over top of the salsa. Serve immediately.

Creamy Cucumber Sandwich

Cucumbers are packed with health benefits. They contain antioxidants, anti-inflammatory, and anti-cancer nutrients as well as vitamin K, molybdenum, pantothenic acid, copper, potassium, manganese, vitamin C, phosphorus, magnesium, biotin, and vitamin B1.

Ingredients

Whole wheat bread.....2 thick slices

Cream cheese, softened.....2 tablespoons

Cucumber.....6 slices

Alfalfa sprouts.....2 tablespoons

Red wine vinegar.....1 teaspoon

Tomato.....1 sliced

Lettuce.....1 leaf (your choice of lettuce)

Pepperoncini.....1 ounce, sliced (yellow sweetly pickled bell peppers)

Avocado..... ½ mashed

Extra virgin olive oil.....1 teaspoon

Directions

Spread one side of each bread slice with softened cream cheese.

Add the cucumber slices and alfalfa sprouts.

Sprinkle with oil then vinegar.

Layer tomato slices, lettuce, and pepperoncini.

Add mashed avocado to the other slice of bread and place on top to complete your cucumber sandwich. Serve.

Pepper Jack Bacon Chicken Sandwich

Pepper-jack cheese is simply Monterey Jack cheese with spicy hot peppers added to it. Usually the jalapeno or habanero pepper is used because of its spicy flavors.

Chicken is a source of high protein. Choose a lean breast that is low in fat and calories. The combination of chicken, bacon, and vegetables makes this sandwich simply delectable!

Ingredients

Bacon.....8 slices

Chicken breast.....4 skinless boneless halves

Poultry seasoning.....2 teaspoons

Pepper Jack cheese.....4 slices

Whole wheat buns.....4 split

Lettuce leaves.....4 (your choice of lettuce)

Tomato.....4 slices

Onions.....½ cup, thinly sliced

Dill pickle.....12 slices

Directions

Light the grill and let it heat up in advance.

In a medium skillet, cook the bacon on the stove over medium high heat until browned on both sides. Remove from the pan and drain on paper towels to reduce the oil content.

Rub the chicken with the poultry seasoning and place on the grill. Cook the chicken for 6 minutes or until it is cooked through.

Top each piece of chicken with 2 slices of bacon and 1 slice of pepper jack cheese.

Continue to grill for 2-3 minutes allowing the cheese to melt evenly.

Place chicken on each bun and add tomato, lettuce, onion, and pickle slices.

Serve immediately.

Beef Broccoli Stir-Fry

The difference between Tamari soy sauce and regular soy sauce is in the wheat to soy ratio. Tamari sauce uses very little wheat and mostly soy, while soy sauce tends to use more wheat. Soy sauce also has a saltier taste.

Serves 2 -3

Ingredients

Coconut oil, butter, or ghee.....2 tablespoons

Minced beef.....500 grams

Garlic.....2 cloves, finely sliced

Broccoli.....2 heads

Tamari soy sauce.....4 tablespoons

Coriander.....1 bunch, chopped

Dried or fresh chili.....to taste (optional)

Fresh ginger..... 2-3 tablespoons, finely shredded (optional)

Roasted cashews.....1 handful, chopped (optional)

Directions

Preheat the wok or skillet on high adding a drizzle of coconut oil

Add the beef and brown it on all sides.

While beef is browning, wash and cut the broccoli into bite-sized chunks.

Add the garlic, chilies, and ginger to the beef then continue to cook until well browned.

Add broccoli and water. Cover the pan and continue to cook for a few minutes stirring periodically. Broccoli should be tender but still holding a crunch.

Season with coriander and serve with cashews on top.

Bruschetta with Tomato, Garlic, and Basil

Bruschetta is an antipasto. Antipasto means "before the meal" in Italy so the antipasto is the first course served in a formal meal. Bruschetta typically includes grilled bread that's been soaked in olive oil then rubbed with garlic, and topped with tomatoes salt, pepper, and a light drizzle of olive oil. This succulent dish is great any time of the day and offers a high level of vitamin C along with a long list of heart-healthy nutrients.

Makes 6 to 10 servings

Ingredients

Ripe plum tomatoes.....6 or 7 (about 1 ½ pounds)

Garlic.....2 cloves, minced

Balsamic vinegar..... 1 teaspoon

Fresh basil leaves.....6-8 chopped

French bread baguette.....1 or a similar Italian bread

Extra virgin olive oil.....¼ cup

Salt and black pepper.....to taste

Directions

Preheat oven to 450 °F (225 °C).

Take the bread and cut it into ½ inch slices, diagonally.

Coat each side of the sliced bread with olive oil using a pastry brush.

Place sliced and brushed bread on a cookie sheet then toast on the top rack of the oven. Watch for the bread to turn brown, about 5 to 6 minutes.

Align the toasted garlic and olive oil bread on a platter making sure the olive oil is facing up.

You can have a tomato based salsa in the platters center bowl, or you can arrange tomatoes around the platter with a serving fork.

You can also place the tomatoes directly on each slice of bread. The bread will get soggy if placed directly on top, so serve immediately in that instance.

Note: If you don't want to use the oven for toasting, you can use a griddle. Start with the sliced bread and toast on the griddle. Use a sharp knife and score the toast then add garlic to the scores and drizzle olive oil on each side using about a teaspoon in total.

Light Lettuce Wraps with Tuna and Avocado

Tuna that is packed in water offers higher nutritional value than tuna that is packed in oil. The cheaper oils used to pack tuna do not have a high nutritional rating and are not necessarily the "tuna oil" itself. Albacore packed in water is a higher quality canned solid tuna that offers more nutrients than regular tuna.

Serves 2

Ingredients

Tuna.....1 can, flaked

Avocado.....½ mashed

Homemade mayonnaise.....2 tablespoons

Green olives.....¼ cup, sliced

Green chili.....2 tablespoons, diced

Scallion.....1 finely sliced

Green leaf lettuce.....2 large leaves (choose your favorite greens)

Homemade mayonnaise:

Egg yolk.....1 large

Fresh lemon juice.....1 ½ teaspoons

White wine vinegar..... 1 teaspoon

Dijon mustard..... ¼ teaspoon

Salt.....½ teaspoon or to taste

Canola oil.....¾ cup, divided

Homemade mayonnaise directions:

Separate the egg whites and yolks. Put the egg yolks in a small mixing bowl and discard the egg whites.

In a small mixing bowl, combine the egg yolk, lemon juice, vinegar, mustard and ½ teaspoon salt. Whisk until the ingredients are blended and become bright yellow.

Add ¼ cup canola oil to the mixture while whisking constantly. Only add a few drops at a time. Add the remaining ½ cup of oil very slowly in a thin stream, whisking constantly until the mayonnaise becomes thick.

Tuna Avocado Lettuce Wrap directions:

Pit and slice the olives in half then set aside.

Finely slice the scallions and set aside.

Use a pair of disposable gloves when cutting chilies. Dice the green chili and set aside. Do not get the chili juice on the counter surface or cross contaminate as the juice from the green chili can cause a burning sensation.

In a small bowl, mash the avocado with a fork until smooth and creamy. Add the chilled mayonnaise and mix until well blended. Add the tuna, olives, scallions, and green chilies to the avocado and mayonnaise mixture. Stir until the ingredients are well coated.

Place one large lettuce leaf on a plate and spoon the tuna salad onto the lettuce leaf. Wrap closed then serve immediately.

Exotic Mango Chicken Lettuce Wraps

Mangos are jam-packed with vitamin A, vitamin C, fiber, and antioxidants. They are an excellent low calorie, low-fat, and cholesterol free snack.

Ingredients

Ground chicken.....1 pound (you can also use ground chicken thighs for more flavor)

Soy sauce.....2 teaspoons

Cornstarch.....1 teaspoon (potato or rice starch are also okay)

Cooking oil.....1 teaspoon (a high smoke point oil would be best such as rice bran oil, grape seed oil, or canola oil)

Green onions.....2 chopped

Shiitake mushrooms.....4 ounces, sliced

Seasoned rice vinegar.....2 teaspoons

Toasted sesame oil..... ½ teaspoon

Mango.....1 large, diced

Bib lettuce.....1 head rinsed, leaves separated

Directions

In a large bowl, add the ground chicken, soy sauce, and cornstarch. Stir to mix and set aside to marinate.

Heat a wok or large skillet to medium heat. When the wok or skillet is hot, add the cooking oil.

Add the green onions and the shiitake mushrooms and cook them for a minute or two.

Increase the heat to high and add the ground chicken, soy sauce, and cornstarch mixture. Stir and break up the chicken to make sure it cooks evenly all the way through, 5-7 minutes.

Add seasoned rice vinegar, sesame oil, and diced mango.

Remove from heat. Adjust seasonings to taste.

Create cups with the lettuce and scoop the chicken mixture into the lettuce. Serve warm.

Options:

Stir in a small spoonful of chili sauce, or add a few chili pepper flakes to the oil as it is heating. Top with some fresh cilantro leaves. Experiment with other meats such as lamb, turkey, beef, or pork. You can also try subbing out the mango with mandarin orange slices.

Chapter 3
DINNER

To keep the body in good health is a duty, otherwise we shall not be able to keep our mind strong and clear.

– Buddha

Cheesy Artichoke Stuffed Chicken Breasts

Artichokes are among the top five highest phytonutrient, antioxidant foods. In fact, artichokes have more antioxidants than any other vegetable. Goat cheese is a wonderful source of protein and probiotics.

Ingredients

Chicken breasts.....2 thinned to 1/8 inch

Light goat cheese.....1 ounce

Artichoke hearts..... ½ cup

Directions

Preheat oven to 375 °F (190 °C).

Place the chicken in a freezer bag and close. Use a kitchen mallet or rolling pin to thin the chicken breasts to 1/8 inches.

In a food processor, add the artichokes and goat cheese then blend until creamy.

Lay the flattened chicken breast onto the baking sheet.

Spoon the artichoke mixture over one side of the chicken then fold the other side over the mixture.

Bake for 15-20 minutes. The cooking time will depend on the size of the chicken breast and the amount of filling. Make sure the chicken is cooked through then serve immediately.

Chicken Cilantro Masala Burgers

Making chicken burgers instead of beef burgers brings a different amount of nutrients to the dinner table. A chicken burger has higher levels of B3, protein, and selenium while beef has higher levels of B12 and B6. Garam Masala is a blend of spices that include turmeric, black and white peppercorns, cloves, cinnamon, black and white cumin seeds, and black, brown and white cardamom pods.

Makes 16 patties

Ingredients

Ground chicken......4 pounds

Cilantro......1 cup

Eggs.....2 large

Garam Masala.....3 tablespoons

Garlic paste.....1 tablespoon

Ginger paste.....1 tablespoon

Scallions.....1 cup, chopped

Serrano peppers.....3 finely chopped

Directions

In a medium bowl, add the chicken, cilantro, eggs, Garam Masala, garlic paste, ginger paste, scallions and the finely chopped Serrano peppers.

Form the mixture into 16 patties.

In a medium skillet, on medium high heat, fry the chicken burgers on both sides until nicely browned.

Cover the skillet with a lid for the last 5 minutes to make sure it cooks through to the center.

Balsamic Lemon-Garlic Salmon

Balsamic vinegar originated in Italy. The cost of balsamic vinegar can vary considerably depending on the quality. The flavor of true balsamic vinegar includes hints of honey, fig, caramel and raisin. It has a smooth taste and can be sipped like a fine port or liqueur. True Aceto balsamic vinegar is aged for a minimum of 10 years and a 3.4 ounce bottle sells from $50-$500.

Ingredients

Sockeye salmon fillets.....8 ounces

Balsamic vinegar.....2 tablespoons

Extra virgin olive oil.....2 tablespoons

Fresh lemon juice.....1 tablespoon

Garlic.....1 clove, minced

Dash of salt

Directions

Preheat the broiler.

In a medium dish, add salt, balsamic vinegar, lemon juice, garlic, and the olive oil. Whisk the ingredients together.

Dip the fish into the mixture and place on a baking sheet.

Make sure the oven rack is 4 inches from the heat source.

Place the fish in the oven and broil 4 to 6 minutes turning midway.

Fish should flake when finished. Serve with balsamic vinegar.

Quiche with Broccoli and Cheddar

Broccoli is a cruciferous vegetable that is an essential part of our diet. Cruciferous vegetables come from the Brassicaceae or cruciferae family and include broccoli, cabbage, cauliflower, cress, kale, bok choy, and similar green leafy vegetables. These vegetables are linked to lowering the risk of cancer and stopping the growth of cancer cells in tumors.

Ingredients

Cheddar cheese.....½ cup, shredded

Half and half cream.....1 ½ cups

Eggs....3 large

Black pepper....¼ teaspoon

Broccoli.....½ cup

Single 9"pie crust.....1 crust

Directions

Preheat the oven to 375 °F (190 °C).

First, prick the pie shell and bake for 10 minutes. Remove from the oven and set on a baking sheet.

Add cheddar cheese and broccoli in layers ending with the cheese.

Add the pepper over the top layer of cheese.

In a medium bowl, add the eggs and cream. Whisk together until well blended then pour over the cheese and broccoli in the pie shell.

Bake until golden brown. You should be able to insert a knife one inch from the edge and have it come out clean.

Roasted Salmon with Garlic and Herbs

Sockeye salmon is found in the northern Pacific ocean. It is a great source of protein and omega-3's. It is also full of antioxidants and contains vitamin B and E, phosphorus, magnesium, zinc, and selenium.

Ingredients

Salt free garlic and herb seasoning.....1 teaspoon

Lemon.....1 ounce

Sockeye salmon.....3 ounces

Directions

Preheat the oven to 400 °F (200°C).

On a baking sheet, place the salmon skin side down.

Sprinkle the salmon with salt free garlic and herb seasoning.

Bake the salmon for 25 minutes.

Salmon should flake when cooked through.

Remove from oven and squeeze lemon juice over the top then plate.

Chicken with Garlic & Fresh Parsley

Pasture raised chicken provides over 97 percent of our daily allowance of vitamin B12, over 70 percent of our daily protein requirement, and over 56 percent of our selenium requirement...all in just one serving!

Ingredients

Chicken breasts.....3 boneless, skinless

Garlic.....2 teaspoons

Flour.....2 tablespoons

Vegetable oil.....2 tablespoons

Butter.....2 tablespoons

Black pepper.....½ teaspoon

Salt.....½ teaspoon

Fresh parsley.....¼ cup

Directions

In a freezer bag, add the flour, salt and pepper. Seal and turn to mix.

Cut the chicken breast into bite-sized cubes and pat dry with paper towels.

Place the chicken in the freezer bag then seal closed. Turn to coat the chicken evenly.

In a medium skillet, add the vegetable oil and heat on medium high heat. Add the chicken to the skillet and cook 3 ½ minutes. Turn while cooking.

Add the garlic, parsley, and butter. Sauté for 1 minute while stirring to coat the chicken. Serve immediately.

Grilled Red Snapper

Red snapper is a great source of omega-3s. The tasty combination of grilled red snapper and tomatoes provides a large dose of heart healthy nutrients that will help you meet your weekly dietary needs.

Ingredients

Extra virgin olive oil....1 tablespoon

Lemon..... ½ squeezed

Garlic..... 3 cloves minced

Cherry tomatoes.....½ cup halved

Red snapper.....6 fillets

Salt.....½ teaspoon

Dash of pepper

Directions

In a small bowl, add the olive oil, lemon juice, and minced garlic then whisk together.

Add the red snapper fillets to the mixture then let it sit for 10 minutes to marinate.

While the fillets are marinating, prepare the grill.

Add the marinated fish to the prepared and heated grill rack. Flip the fish over after about 5 minutes.

The fish should be completely cooked within 10 minutes. Plate and serve immediately.

Seared Tuna and Parmesan with Shaved Fennel Salad

There is nothing like the great taste of tuna paired with parmesan. This recipe calls for sushi grade tuna. Tuna is a nutrient dense fish. It is an excellent source of protein, selenium, magnesium, potassium, vitamin B6, vitamin B12, niacin, folic acid, and the most beneficial omega-3 fatty acids.

Ingredients

Boneless sushi grade tuna.....4 ounces

Parmesan cheese.....2 tablespoons

Fresh parsley.....1 teaspoon

Pink peppercorns.....1 tablespoon

Fresh thyme leaves..... 1/8 teaspoon

Salt.....¼ teaspoon

Extra virgin olive oil.....1 ½ teaspoons

Lemon juice..... ½ ounce (2 tablespoons)

Fennel bulb.....1 shaved paper thin

Directions

Salad:

In a medium bowl, add fennel, oil, lemon juice, parsley, thyme, and parmesan cheese. Set aside.

Tuna:

In a medium skillet on high heat, add the olive oil and allow it to heat.

Add the tuna and cook for 30 seconds. Turn and cook the other side for another 30 seconds then remove from heat.

Cut tuna into five slices.

Plating:

Using a serving platter, add the fennel salad and place the five slices of tuna fish toward the center of the platter on top of the salad. Serve immediately.

Crème Fraîche Prawns with Green Peppercorns

The name Crème fraîche means "fresh cream." It is a soured cream that contains 30 to 40 percent butterfat and mostly resembles sour cream or yogurt though its flavor is much richer and its texture is much creamier. Crème fraîche is widely used in French cooking.

Ingredients

Crème Fraîche..... 2 ounces

Green peppercorns.....2 tablespoons

Extra virgin olive oil.....1 tablespoon

Shallots.....3 tablespoons, chopped

Dry white wine.....6 fluid ounces

Prawns.....1 pound, large

Directions

In a large saucepan on medium low heat, add the olive oil and chopped shallots. Sauté the shallots until lightly browned. Add white wine and simmer for 3 minutes.

Add the prawns and cook on high heat for 5 minutes. Remove the prawns from the pan and set them aside.

Add peppercorns to the cooking sauce and reduce the volume of the sauce by half. Lower the heat and add crème fraîche. Cook for 2 minutes.

Return the prawns to the pan and heat gently. Remove the prawns and sauce from saucepan and serve.

Turkey Meatball Mini's

Turkey meatballs are a great way to cut some of the fat associated with beef. By substituting turkey for beef you lose the fat but not the flavor. This mini meatball is packed with flavor! Turkey is a great source of niacin and selenium. It is also lower in calories than beef.

Ingredients

Parmesan cheese.....2 tablespoons, grated

Egg.....1 large

Black pepper.....1 teaspoon

Fresh basil.....5 leaves, chopped

Salt.....1 teaspoon

Ground turkey.....1 ½ pounds

Garlic.....1 clove, chopped

Yellow onion.....¼ cup, chopped

Extra virgin olive oil.....2 tablespoons

Directions

In a medium bowl, add the parmesan cheese, egg, pepper, chopped basil, salt, ground turkey, garlic, and chopped onions.

Heat the olive oil in a medium skillet on medium heat.

While the oil is heating, go back to the medium bowl and mix the ingredients well, then form small balls.

Put the meatballs in the heated oil and brown on all sides. Let them cook through.

Serve the mini meatballs with marinara sauce on pasta or in a sub sandwich with mozzarella cheese on top.

Black Bean Chili

Black beans provide a high level of molybdenum, folate, fiber, and copper among other nutrients. They help the digestive tract move food which helps steady the digestive process. This helps to lessen the strain on the digestive tract while supporting an optimal chemical balance from the food we eat.

Ingredients

Chili seasoning mix.....9 grams

Diced tomatoes with green chilies.....15 ounces

Black beans.....31 ounces

Lean ground beef.....1 pound

Directions

In a large iron skillet, crumble and cook the beef until nicely browned.

Drain the fat from the skillet.

Add diced tomatoes with green chilies, black beans, and chili seasoning. Stir all the ingredients together.

Simmer for 20-25 minutes and serve warm.

Grilled Cinnamon and Coriander Lamb Chops

Grass-fed lamb chops provide over 104 percent of our daily recommended value for B12. They also provide over 51 percent of our daily recommended value for protein and half of our recommended daily values for selenium and vitamin B3, which we often lack in our weekly vitamin intake.

Ingredients

Ground cinnamon.....1 tablespoon

Ground coriander..... 1 tablespoon

Lamb chops.....1 pound

Directions

Preheat the broiler or grill to medium heat. Place the lamb chops on a baking pan and brush with water.

Sprinkle the cinnamon and coriander over the lamb chops and then rub the seasonings into the lamb chops to ensure the flavors infuse the meat.

Grill or broil the lamb chops turning them over periodically. Cook 20 minutes or until done.

Pecan and Parmesan Pork Chops

This recipe is a great way to get protein and good fat in one dish. Pecans are an excellent source of energy and contain a wealth of nutrients, minerals, antioxidants, and vitamins that are necessary for good health. They are rich in monounsaturated fatty acids that help decrease bad cholesterol and increase good cholesterol in the blood. Pecans are also a wonderful source of vitamin-E and contain rich sources of B-complex groups of vitamins. Eat a handful of pecans a day to maintain great health.

Ingredients

Egg whites.....2 from two large eggs

Pecan nuts.....1 cup, finely chopped

Pork chops.....4-10 ounce pork chops, thick cut, bone-in

Parmesan cheese.....½ cup, shredded

Black pepper.....1 teaspoon

Salt.....1 teaspoon

Directions

Trim any separable fat off the pork chops.

Mix the pecans and parmesan cheese together.

Place the egg whites in a shallow dish.

Pour the pecan and parmesan cheese mixture into a separate shallow dish.

Dip the pork chops in the egg whites then roll them in the pecan cheese mix.

Place them on a sprayed 9x13 pan. Lightly place some tin foil over the pork chops and bake at 375°F (190 °C) for 25 minutes.

Remove the tin foil and bake another 5 minutes more. Serve.

Jambalaya

Shrimp is loaded with vitamin D, protein, zinc, and vitamin B3. It is a wonderful carbohydrate-free food for anyone interested in losing weight.

Ingredients

Garlic......3 teaspoons, minced

Green onions.....3 small young green onions

Black beans.....½ cup

Raw shrimp.....12 ounces without shell

Cajun spices.....buy premade or make your own below

White rice.....2 cups precooked (can use brown rice if preferred)

Polish sausage.....14 ounces, cooked

Celery.....1 cup, chopped

Cajun Spice:

Salt.....2 teaspoons

Garlic powder......2 teaspoons

Paprika.....2½ teaspoons

Black pepper.....1 teaspoon

Onion powder.....1 teaspoon

Cayenne pepper.....1 teaspoon

Dried oregano.....1 ¼ teaspoons

Red pepper.....½ teaspoon

Cajun spice directions:

Add all the ingredients to a small plastic bowl with a tight fitting lid.

Shake the ingredients together and use as needed.

Directions

Precooked Rice:

If you do not have precooked rice on hand then prepare 2 cups of rice with 4 cups of water. Rice is always cooked as one part rice to two parts water.

Boil the water, add the rice and simmer for 5 minutes while the rice returns to a boil. Be sure to stir the rice since it will stick to the bottom if you don't.

When the rice water is boiling, reduce the heat to simmer and place a tight fitting lid on the pot. Most rice will cook through within 15 minutes.

If cooking brown rice you may need to cook longer, so check the package directions to confirm cooking times.

Main course:

In a large skillet, add the green onions, celery, and garlic. Sauté.

Stir in the precooked Polish sausage and raw shrimp.

Add the Cajun spice to taste.

Sauté the ingredients for another 5 minutes.

Stir to mix all the ingredients together well

Add the rice and black beans.

Cook for another 5-10 minutes until all the ingredients cook through and have absorbed the Cajun flavors. Serve warm.

Mexican Shrimp Pasta

Ancho is the name used for a type of dried chili pepper most commonly used in Mexican cooking. The ancho chili is a dried Pablano pepper. Anchos have a sweet, smoky flavor similar to raisins. They have a deep red color, a wrinkled skin and their heat level is between mild to medium-hot.

Ingredients

Spaghetti or fettuccini..... 8 ounces

Vegetable, grape seed, or canola oil..... ½ cup

Garlic.....3 cloves, thinly sliced

Ancho chilies.....1 ounce (about 2 medium to large) dried, rinsed, seeded, and deveined

Raw shrimp.....½ pound (21-25 count) peeled, deveined, and tails removed, cut the shrimp pieces into thirds

Parmesan cheese..... freshly grated

Lime or lemon juice.....freshly squeezed

Salt.....to taste

Black pepper.....to taste

Directions

Sauce:

In a large skillet on medium high heat, add the oil and garlic. Brown the sliced garlic on both sides and remove from the skillet with a slotted spoon. Put the browned garlic in a large bowl and set aside.

While the garlic is cooking, using disposable gloves, slice the ancho chilies then seed and rinse them. Roll them up and cut them into slices.

When garlic is done add the ancho chilies to the oil and cook for half a minute then remove with a slotted spoon, draining the oil back into the skillet. Do not overcook in order to avoid bitter chilies. Put the chilies in a large bowl with the browned garlic

Pasta:

In a large pot ¾ full of water, add salt and cook on high heat to get water boiling for pasta.

When water begins to boil, add the pasta and cook to al dente (firm to bite).

Strain the pasta when cooked and add to the large bowl of garlic, and chilies.

Putting it all together:

Add the shrimp to the skillet and increase the heat to high.

Cook the shrimp until it turns pink. Stir constantly to prevent burning.

When cooked through, remove from heat and pour the shrimp along with the oil into the large bowl with the garlic and chilies.

Stir to combine all the ingredients. Serve warm with parmesan, salt and pepper.

Cod Fish Cakes

Cod is fantastic for providing over 109 percent of our B12 daily intake values. And that's by eating only one serving of cod. Cod belongs to the same family of fish as haddock and pollock. It is an excellent low-calorie source of protein containing 21 grams of protein in a 4oz serving. It also contains a variety of important nutrients that help maintain good health.

Ingredients

Cod fillets.....1 pound

Russet potatoes.....2 medium-sized

Bread crumbs..... 1 cup

Fresh parsley..... ¼ cup, chopped

Parmesan cheese.....2 tablespoons, freshly grated

Garlic.....2 cloves, finely chopped

Salt and pepper.....1 teaspoon each

Eggs.....2 lightly beaten

Grape seed or canola oil

Directions

Mashed Potatoes:

Peel the potatoes. Cut them into quarters and add them to a large pot of boiling water.

Cook for about 20 minutes on high heat.

Strain the water. Place potatoes into a medium to large bowl.

Mash the potatoes with a potato masher or electric mixer. Set aside.

Cod:

Broil cod 4 inches from the broiler until the tops of the cod are brown.

Turn them over and broil until the cod flakes.

Remove from broiler and add them to the potatoes, breaking up the cod into pieces as they are added to the potatoes.

Cod Fish Cakes:

Take the bowl of potatoes and cod and add breadcrumbs, parsley, parmesan cheese, salt, pepper, and garlic.

Stir the ingredients together to mix well.

Add the two eggs one at a time.

Stir the mixture between adding eggs.

In a medium skillet, heat the grape seed or canola oil to medium high heat. Drop a small piece of the cod mixture into the oil. If it sizzles, the oil is ready for cooking.

Take a large spoonful of the cod mixture and form patties. Carefully place each patty in the skillet of hot oil. Continue to form patties and place them in the skillet.

Allow the patties to brown on one side then turn them over and allow them to brown on the other side cooking them through.

Remove from skillet and place on a plate of paper towels to draw the oil out.

Transfer to serving platter and serve immediately.

Cod Poached in Court Bouillon

Court Bouillon is a rich flavored liquid that is used to cook fish, seafood, vegetables, eggs, sweetbreads, and delicate meats. Traditionally court bouillon has been used to poach seafood. The name "court bouillon" means short, briefly boiled broth because it only cooks for a short time compared to other more complex stock.

Ingredients

Poached Cod:

Water.....2 quarts

Salt.....1 tablespoon

Garlic.....2 cloves, crushed

Bay leaves.....2

Extra virgin olive oil..... 1 tablespoon

Cod fillets.....2 pounds (or other firm white fish, not sole), cut to fit the pan

Lemon.....for garnish

Optional side of saffron potatoes:

Yukon gold potatoes.....1 pound, cut into 1 ½ - inch chunks (peel on or off, your choice)

Saffron..... pinch

Salt.....to taste

Directions

Court Bouillon:

In a large saucepan, add 2 quarts of water, salt, garlic, olive oil, and bay leaves. Cook on high heat for up to 10 minutes ensuring the water gets infused with the garlic and bay leaf flavors.

Additional ingredients such as celery, white wine, lemon juice, and thyme are terrific additions and offer different variations of court bouillon.

Poached Cod:

Rinse the cod fillets and place them in the court bouillon. Let the liquid return to a simmering boil. This should take 2-4 minutes.

When the liquid is at a simmering boil, let the fish cook an additional 2-3 minutes depending on the size of the fillets.

Remove the cod from the liquid and cover with foil while preparing potatoes. Keep the court bouillon liquid. You will need it for the potatoes.

Saffron Potatoes:

Add a pinch of saffron to the court bouillon and let the water boil.

Wash the potatoes, cut them into chunks then add them to the court bouillon with saffron seasoning.

Simmer for 15-20 minutes. When the potatoes are ready, you will be able to pierce them with a fork. Remove the potatoes with a slotted spoon and plate them with the poached cod.

Season with additional salt if desired then serve hot.

Ground Turkey Garam Masala with Potatoes

The word Garam is a Hindi word that means hot. Masala means spices. Put them together and you get some hot mixed spices for this ground turkey with potatoes meal!

Turmeric which is used to make curry is from the mustard family and offers a long list of health benefits along with its spicy flavor. Turmeric is also excellent for heart health, cancer prevention, and rheumatoid arthritis. It also reduces the risk of childhood leukemia and improves liver function. These are just some of the many benefits of turmeric.

Ingredients

Vegetable oil..... 3-4 tablespoons

Ground turkey..... 1 pound (thigh meat is preferred)

Yellow onion.....1 chopped

Garlic.....2 cloves, chopped

Fresh red chilies..... 1-2 chopped

Ginger.....1-inch, peeled, finely grated

Water.....½ cup

Salt.....to taste

Garam Masala..... 1 tablespoon

Turmeric..... 1 teaspoon

Cumin..... 1 teaspoon

Ground coriander..... 1 teaspoon

Yukon Gold potatoes.....2 large peeled and cut into 1-inch chunks

Roma or other plum tomatoes..... 2-4 diced

Fresh or frozen peas..... 1 cup

Fresh cilantro or parsley.....½ cup, chopped

Directions

In a medium skillet on medium high heat, add the oil and ground turkey.

Let the turkey brown and simmer without stirring.

When browned, add the onion and chilies to the ground turkey.

Sauté the mixture until the onions begin to turn opaque.

Add the salt and stir

Add the grated ginger and garlic to the mixture and stir.

Sauté another 2 minutes to infuse with flavors.

Add the turmeric, cumin, coriander, ½ cup of water and potatoes.

Stir the ingredients together and mix well.

Turn the heat down to a medium low simmer for 15 minutes or until the potatoes are tender

Add the diced tomatoes and peas. Mix them together well with the potato mixture. Cover and cook for an additional 2-3 minutes adding salt if needed.

Add cilantro before serving. This dish is great with wild rice or a flatbread.

Chapter 4
DESSERTS

Looking after my health today gives me a better hope for tomorrow.

– Anne Wilson Shaef

Sugar Free Banana Cookies

Bananas are a great source of potassium. Their health benefits include maintaining normal blood pressure and heart function, and protection from ulcers. They also support eye and kidney health and promote strong bones.

Ingredients

Bananas.....3 ripe, medium

Rolled oats.....2 cups

Dates.....1 cup, pitted and chopped

Vegetable oil.....1/3 cup

Vanilla extract.....1 teaspoon

Directions

Preheat oven to 350°F (175 °C)

In a large bowl, add the bananas and mash with a fork.

Add the vanilla extract, dates, oil, and rolled oats.

Mix the ingredients together well.

To form the cookies use two tablespoons. Fill one tablespoon full of dough then push the dough off that spoon onto an ungreased cookie sheet with the second spoon.

Bake for 20 minutes or until lightly brown.

Sugarless Pumpkin Pie

Canned pumpkin contains fiber, vitamin A, vitamin E, and iron? Canned pumpkin is different from the canned pumpkin pie mixes that contain sugar. It can be added to soups as a tasty thickener, to oatmeal, shakes, wraps, omelets, dressings and a number of other foods to jazz up the flavors.

Ingredients

9-inch baked pie shell.....1 shell

Sugar free instant vanilla pudding..... 2 small boxes

Milk.....2 cups

Plain canned pumpkin.....2 cups (not pumpkin pie mixture)

Nutmeg.....¼ teaspoon

Ginger.....¼ teaspoon

Cinnamon..... ½ teaspoon

Directions

In a large bowl, mix the instant vanilla pudding, milk, canned pumpkin, nutmeg, ginger, and cinnamon. You can mix with an electric mixer or put right in the blender.

Mix the ingredients until smooth.

Pour into the pie shell and refrigerate.

Raspberry Coconut Ripple

Raspberries have long been associated with cancer prevention. Their phytonutrients play a huge role in reducing inflammation and altering the reproduction of cancer cells. New studies show positive signs that raspberries may actually change the signals that are sent to potential or existing cancer cells instructing them to include cell death as a cycle. Raspberries also include a wealth of vitamins and minerals essential for good health. They can also help alleviate arthritis and assist in weight loss.

Serves 6-8

Ingredients

Frozen raspberries..... 1/3 cup

Shredded coconut..... 1/3 cup

Coconut oil..... 1/3 cup

Organic, salted butter..... 80 grams

Raw cacao powder or cocoa..... 2 tablespoons

Rice malt syrup..... 2 tablespoons

Directions

Line a dinner plate with wax paper.

Scatter the berries and shredded coconut on the plate.

In a small saucepan, melt the butter and oil.

Stir in the raw cacao powder, or cocoa, and rice malt syrup.

Stir until the syrup melts and the mixture blends smoothly.

Pour the smooth mixture over the berries and coconut.

Put into the freezer for 20 minutes or until firm.

Break or cut into shards and serve immediately.

Apple and Oatmeal Cookies

Apples contain wonderful benefits for the cardiovascular system and blood sugar. They also contain essential antioxidants and aid in lowering the risk of lung cancer. Apples also boost your immune system, lower cholesterol, decrease the risk of diabetes and support brain health.

Ingredients

Margarine..... ½ cup, softened

Honey.....½ cup

Egg.....1 medium or large

Vanilla extract..... 1 teaspoon

Whole wheat flour..... ¾ cup, stone ground

Whole Baking soda..... ½ teaspoon

Ground cinnamon..... ¾ teaspoon

Quick cooking oats..... 1 ½ cups

Apple.....1 cored and chopped (any kind)

Directions

Preheat oven to 375°F (190°C).

Grease cookie sheets.

In a medium bowl, add the margarine, eggs, honey, and vanilla. Beat until smooth.

In a large bowl, add the whole-wheat flour, cinnamon, and baking soda. Use a sifter to mix and fluff the ingredients.

Add the creamy mixture to the dry mixture and stir them together.

Add the oats and then the apple and stir until well mixed.

Drop by teaspoonfuls onto the prepared cookie sheets.

Bake 8-10 minutes.

Allow cookies to cool on wire rack for 5 minutes before serving warm.

Sugar Free Chocolate Ice Cream

The difference between plain yogurt and Greek yogurt is the amount of times it gets strained and how much liquid remains after the straining process is completed. One of the best health benefits of Greek yogurt is the probiotics that it offers.

Ingredients

Plain gelatin.....1 teaspoon, plain

Milk.....2 ½ cups, low fat

Sugar Free chocolate drink mix.....½ cup (I would recommend using Nestle)

Plain Greek yogurt..... 1 cup

Vanilla extract..... 1 teaspoon

Dash of salt

Ice cream maker

Directions

In a small saucepan on medium high heat, add one half cup of milk and gelatin. Stir until the gelatin dissolves in the milk then remove from heat.

While the gelatin is dissolving, fill the kitchen sink with enough cold water to submerge the saucepan halfway, allowing the gelatin contents to cool quickly to room temperature.

Pour the cooled gelatin into a blender or food processor. Add the remaining milk, yogurt, vanilla, milk chocolate mix, and salt to the gelatin mixture and blend until smooth.

Cover and chill in the refrigerator until ready to freeze.

Blend for a few seconds before pouring into the ice cream maker.

Follow the ice cream maker's directions from this point forward.

Jell-O Raspberry Whip

Jell-O contains collagen which is the material that makes up bone and cartilage. It also plays a role in weight loss, arthritis prevention, healing brittle bones, and strengthening nails, and joints.

Ingredients

Sour cream.....2 cups

Raspberry sugar free Jell-o.....2 packages

Water.....2 cups

Directions

Fill a medium saucepan with two cups of water and bring it to a boil.

Add the packages of Jell-O to the boiling water and let the Jell-O dissolve.

Using a hand whisk, slowly whisk in the sour cream until well mixed.

Pour into cups, cover with plastic wrap, and refrigerate.

Peanut Butter Mousse

Organic peanut butter can reduce the risk of cardiovascular disease as well as stroke. It also helps to reduce the development of gallstones.

Serves 2

Ingredients

Cottage cheese..... 250 grams

Smooth peanut butter..... 1 ½ tablespoons

Granulated Stevia..... 1 teaspoon

Directions

Place the cottage cheese, peanut butter, and Stevia in a high powered blender.

Pulse until the cottage cheese lumps are gone and the mixture is smooth.

You may need a splash of water while blending to help smooth the ingredients together.

When mixed and smooth, divide the ingredients into two glasses and place in the freezer for 10 minutes.

Chia Seed Power Balls

Chia seeds provide a huge amount of nutrients with virtually zero calories. They are loaded with antioxidants and contain high levels of quality protein and fiber that can help you lose weight. Chia seeds are also a great source of omega-3. They reduce inflammation; enhance cognitive performance and lower cholesterol. They are also a source of calcium, phosphorus, magnesium, and manganese.

Makes 10 power balls

Ingredients

Sweet potatoes..... 450 grams cooked and mashed

Almond butter....2 heaping tablespoons

Chia seeds..... 1 tablespoon

Raw cacao powder.....2 teaspoons

Ground cinnamon.....1 teaspoon

Ground ginger..... ¼ teaspoon

Ground cardamom..... ¼ teaspoon

Ground liquorice..... ¼ teaspoon

Coconut oil

Desiccated coconut for rolling

Directions

In a large bowl, combine the mashed sweet potatoes, almond butter, and Chia seeds.

In a small bowl, mix the cacao powder, cinnamon, ginger, cardamom, and ground liquorice.

Stir the spices from the small bowl into the large bowl of mashed sweet potatoes. Mixing the ingredients together will make the dough gooey and sticky.

In a small bowl, add a few drops of the coconut oil. Dip your fingers into the coconut oil and rub over your hands lightly. Roll the dough into ten balls and chill in the refrigerator for about 20 minutes. Remove from fridge and roll in the desiccated coconut before serving.

The power balls will keep well if refrigerated. Be sure to store in the fridge.

Chocolate Lover's Delight

Cacao is a bean used to make chocolate and cocoa powder. These beans grow on small evergreen trees in Mexico and South America. You can eat cacao beans as a whole bean, broken down into nibs, or ground into powder. Cacao beans are packed with antioxidants, magnesium, and iron.

Serves 2

Ingredients

Mixed berries..... ½ cup, frozen

Avocado..... ½ medium ripe

Baby spinach.....1 cup

Cacao powder..... ¼ cup

Granulated Stevia....½ teaspoon

Vanilla powder.....pinch

Ice cubes..... 2 trays

Directions

In a blender, add the frozen berries, avocado, spinach, cacao powder, granulated stevia, vanilla, and ice cubes.

Blend all the ingredients on high speed and pour into bowls immediately. Serve cold.

You can also pour into ice cube trays and freeze for a hot day when you want a bit of cold chocolate.

Sugar Free Peanut Butter Cups

There is nothing like a little peanut butter to go with the wonderful flavor of chocolate. Yum! Peanuts and cacao powder contain high amounts of antioxidants. Put them together and POW, you are fighting disease with a terrific tasty treat. These chocolate peanut butter cups are just like the store bought ones ...only way healthier!

Makes 20-25

Ingredients

Coconut oil.....½ cup, melted

Raw cacao powder..... ½ cup

Rice malt syrup..... 1 tablespoon

Coconut cream..... 2 tablespoons (the more you use, the harder the chocolate texture)

Smooth natural peanut butter..... ¼ cup

Sea salt.....large pinch

Chocolate wrappers.....these are the brown wrappers that cover chocolate bars. You can buy mini's for your peanut butter cups.

Directions

In a medium bowl, add the coconut oil and cacao powder.

Mix the ingredients together then add the rice malt syrup and coconut cream.

On a small tray, arrange the chocolate wrappers.

Pour a thin layer of the chocolate mixture into the chocolate wrappers then freeze for 5-10 minutes.

Be sure keep this treat cold or it will melt.

Berry Cobbler

Blackberries are among the highest fiber content plants in the world. They contain antioxidants that reduce inflammation, destroy free radicals, prevent cancer, provide cardiovascular benefits, support eye health, skin health, and digestive tract health. They also prevent diabetes and support bone health.

Blueberries contain a high level of antioxidants that improve memory, support brain health, and benefit the nervous system.

Ingredients

Blueberry syrup..... ½ cup

Cornstarch..... 3 tablespoons

Water..... 3 tablespoons

Cinnamon..... ¾ teaspoon

Blackberries, raspberries or blueberries..... 4 cups

Dough:

Unbleached flour..... 1 cup

Baking powder..... 1 ½ teaspoons

Salt.....½ teaspoon

Margarine..... 2 tablespoons, melted

Apple juice concentrate..... 2 tablespoons

Low fat cherry yogurt..... ¼ cup

Dough directions:

Using a sifter over a large bowl, add the flour, baking powder and salt.

Sift the ingredients.

In a medium bowl, add the margarine, juice concentrate and yogurt.

Mix the ingredients together until smooth.

Pour this mixture into the sifted mixture (in the large bowl) while gently blending with a fork.

Knead for 20-30 seconds then press the dough on a floured surface until it is large enough to cover the deep-dish pie pan.

Directions

Preheat oven to 400°F (200°C).

Use a deep dish pie pan and spray with non-stick spray then set aside.

In a small bowl, add cornstarch and water.

Mix until the cornstarch dissolves in the water.

Add the syrup and cinnamon.

Stir the contents together then set aside.

Rinse the berries and fold into the syrup and cornstarch mixture then pour into the greased deep-dish pie pan.

Place the dough over the berries in the deep-dish pie pan and press the dough against the sides.

Use a fork or knife and poke holes in the middle of the pie to allow it to vent while baking.

Reduce the preheated oven to 375°F (190°C).

Bake the pie for 20 to 25 minutes or until the crust is a light brown.

Other books by Gina Crawford

Sugar Detox for Beginners

Mediterranean Diet for Beginners

Mediterranean Diet Cookbook

DASH Diet for Beginners

DASH Diet Recipes

Paleo for Beginners

5:2 Diet for Beginners

5:2 Diet Recipes

Available on Amazon

Conclusion

I pour my heart into every book I write and make every effort to help you achieve your diet and health goals.

Whether you're interested in living a sugar free life, maintaining a limited sugar lifestyle, or overcoming sugar addiction, I hope these recipes will help you get exactly what you want.

Enjoy!

About Gina Crawford

Understanding what it takes to live a healthy lifestyle, eat right, achieve your goal weight, and love your life shouldn't be complicated. Your time is valuable and the last thing you need is to tackle a 300 page book on how to get your health, weight, and life on track. If you're like most people, you just want the facts in bite-sized, easy to understand pieces that you can apply to your life TODAY!

My name is Gina Crawford. I am a health and "all things natural" enthusiast, author, mother, and wife. Years ago I was overweight, exhausted, unhappy, and desperately aching for a better life. One day, gruelingly tired of my situation, I started researching everything I could on health and transforming my life. I often felt overwhelmed by the amount of information and the changes I had to make, but I persevered and managed to turn my life around one book and one bite at a time.

Now I'm determined to share what I've learned in an easy, non-overwhelming, no fluff, no filler, straight to the point kind of way that will allow others to achieve maximum results in a short amount of time.

I am passionate about every book I write and my goal with each book is to make it simple and concise, yet power-packed with the necessary information you need to transform your life. I have learned first-hand the incredible value of healing ourselves with natural organic foods, natural remedies, exercise, and a positive mindset.

When I'm not writing, I love spending time with my family, cooking, walking, biking, and reading.

My hope is that my books will help you live a healthier, better, more passionate, alive life!

Happy reading!

Made in the USA
Lexington, KY
04 February 2017